WILD NAKED LADIES: Mother Nature's Design for Birth
© 2013 Diana Paul

Diana Paul
415~847~6252 PST 9am to 7pm
Diana@LoveDelivers.org

FIRST EDITION

Cover Photo: Richard James Lee, Devonshire, Bermuda
Designed by Erin Sutherland, Petaluma, California
Joanne's Print Shop, Sausalito, California

ISBN 978-1-4675-5009-3

Paul, Diana
BIRTH DAY   DVD
MISS MARGARET - DVD
FIVE COUNTRIES, SIX BIRTHS, SEVEN BABIES - DVD
ATTENDING BIRTH - DVD
Available at LoveDelivers.org

Wild Naked Ladies: Mother Nature's Design for Birth is companion to the DVD
Five Countries, Six Births, Seven Babies. This video shows women following their
instincts to give birth without interference, without drugs and at home.

For Daniel, Jonathan, Arian, Brian and Maggy
"I love you more!"

Advance Praise from Recent Womb Graduates:

Henry Bleckinger ~ 7 ½ months ~ ate this book up with a smile that said, "Scrumptious!" His mother said, "I can't believe how long he's sitting still!"

James Geller ~ 23 months ~ "Baby, ohhh…"

Quinn A. ~ 26 months ~ read it "Again…Again…Again!"

Ivan Pietro ~ age 3 ~ "Babies are cool"

Amalia Lansing ~ age 5 ~ "I learned lots of things…It made me feel like not having a baby because you have to take care of it for a long time."

Elizabeth Schmalensee ~ 29 ~ "This beautiful, inspiring book brought tears to my eyes. What a loving celebration of the sacred nature of unhindered birth."

Henry David Thoreau ~ 186 ~ "…all good things are wild and free." We believe Henry would have loved this book.

Naked Ladies: Hardy, Sun Loving Belladonna Lilies

Wild Naked Ladies: Women Giving Birth Enthusiastically

"Consider the lilies of the field, how they grow: they labour not, neither do they spin." – Matthew 6:28

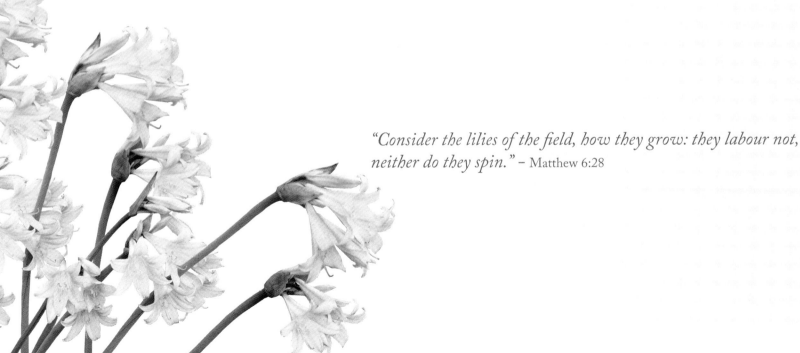

Wild Naked Ladies

Mother Nature's Design For Birth

Diana Paul

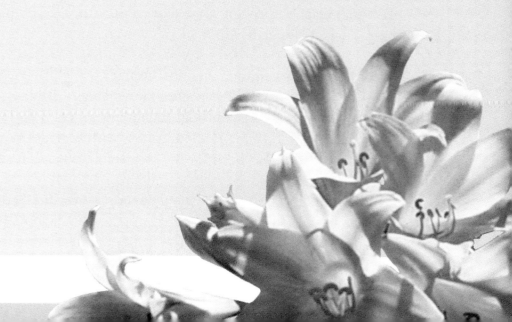

Wildness means following the growth of love.
– Alice Walker

This is an alphabet book about birth. It is another way to share gorgeous images of mothers and babies at work; a truly unique work experienced in one way or another by everyone on the planet. For years, I have explored the transforming power of birth by producing films, speaking, holding film festivals and writing. I am deeply indebted to the mothers and families who share their images and stories with me. Our desires are the same, to elevate consciousness around birth and encourage trust in Mother Nature's design.

In *The Same River Twice*, Alice Walker writes that the message of nature, the universe, the earth and the human heart is "Love. Wildness. And to me, Wildness means following the growth of love. Life is a plant that reaches through stone toward the sun." Reaching "through stone toward the sun," is one of the things "naked lady" (Beladonna Lily) flowers and women giving birth have in common.

I discovered their commonality one summer while driving a friend to town. Just past the stop sign at Las Lomas, I saw a mass of lilies peering down at us. "Oh look at the naked ladies!" I exclaimed stopping the car. Ed whipped his 91 year old head around so fast I had to laugh. "Where?" he queried. "Right there," I said backing up the car. Hundreds of sweetly fragrant flowers danced above us like a chorus waiting to be noticed. If it hadn't been for the stop sign, we wouldn't have seen them.

Later, story poles went up and a bulldozer ran over the "ladybulbs." I winced. Bottles and trash began to accumulate. Blackberry vines started to take over. I thought about rescuing them under cover of night but I didn't have the nerve. I wondered if they would survive.

Wild Naked Ladies

Construction finally ended. August arrived and masses of wild naked ladies trumpeted their indestructibility with another brilliant show. From crushed and broken bulbs, delicate, pink flowers grew right through hard packed dirt toward the sun.

It seems to me that the bulldozer and the naked ladies never should have met. It was a needless clash between high tech and nature. Does this sound at all like birth where nature's design is set aside and bulldozers of fear precede drugs and high tech procedures? Mothers and babies survive, but were all of those interventions necessary?

As a system in the natural universe, birth operates without words or waste. Bulbs and babies don't ask for directions. They grow toward the light. Mothers, hearing their own instincts, know what to trust, when to push, how to surrender. From beginning to end, birth is part of Mother Nature's divinely loving design. It is Her protocols we must obey.

There are billions and billions of birth stories, each one unique. I offer these notes and photos as encouragement and inspiration for reducing the cultural fear and ignorance surrounding birth. Please welcome them and enjoy what is wild, natural and full of love.

Diana Paul

Las Lomas sign surrendering to wild grapes

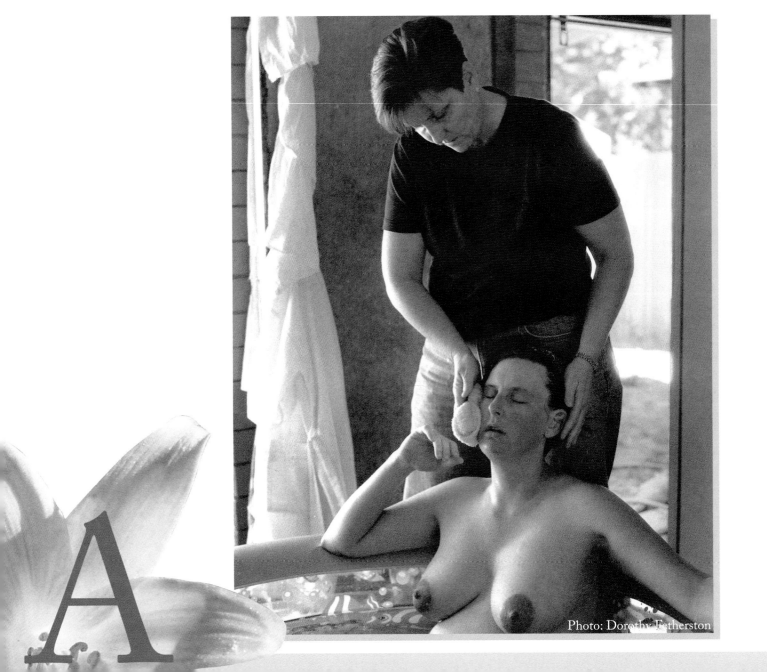

A

Photo: Dorothy Fetherston

Attending

When we interviewed Dr. Marsden Wagner, the cameraman asked, "So Dr. Wagner, when was the last time you delivered a baby?"

We watched Dr. Wagner as he rose up out of his seat, eyes direct and blazing, voice loud and firm, "Doctors don't deliver babies," he said, "WOMEN deliver babies!!!"

Frank drew in his breath and looked at me with a smile. "What a great sound bite," he said.

Getting this concept clear, that "women deliver babies," and everyone else attends, might just renew an old paradigm.

Marsden Wagner, M.D., M.S. is former Director of Women's and Children's Health for the World Health Organization.

A

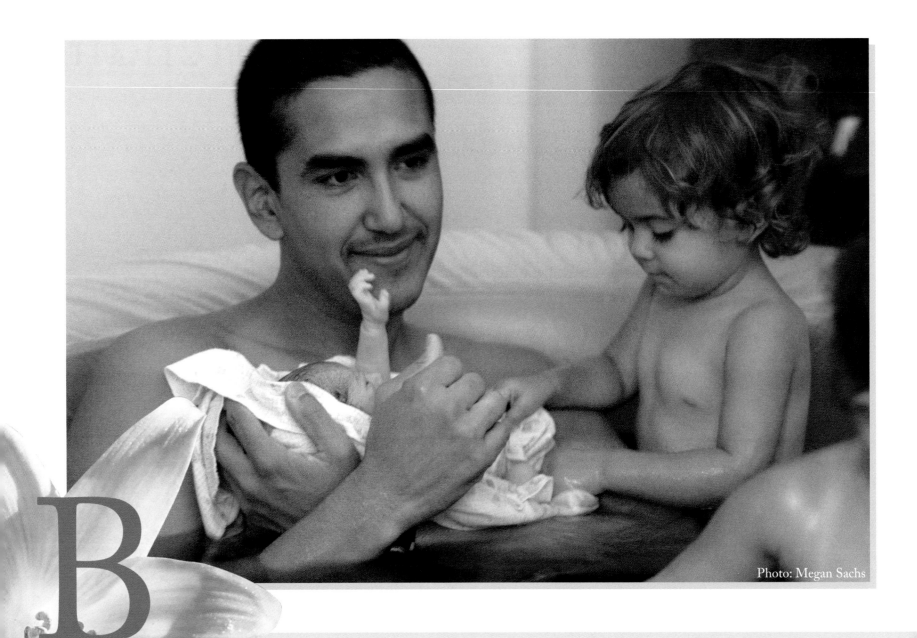

B

Bonding

The baby really belongs to the family. We recommend that the first hour and a quarter belong to the parents. The bath can wait for a couple or three days since the baby is covered with a protective coat. You don't have to rush. And maybe the mother can place him on her chest skin to skin where he gains a great deal of heat. We used to use an incubator to warm up the baby. The mother is faster at reheating the baby and when she reaches the right temperature she turns off her heater and cools the baby. Now the father also heats the baby but he doesn't have a cooling mechanism. So the mother is amazingly connected to her baby. And she's connected with all sorts of mechanisms that she may not know about.

The baby will crawl to the breast. The breasts contain amniotic fluid and if you've not rubbed any of the amniotic fluid off his hands, he will go towards the breast. If you put him in the middle, he will choose which breast to go on. If you don't even touch him except on his bottom, he will kick you on the lower abdomen and that will stimulate uterine contractions and cut down the bleeding. And then he will very, very slowly move to one side or the other, taking time out to rest, taking time out to suck on his hands. They remind him of the nipple. He will slowly go to one side or the other. Before he goes on, he will slowly rub the nipple and elongate it. This allows him to go on the breast easier and suck. It's a very, very interesting phenomenon. Then he will look at the mother's face and he will look right into her eyes and then he will connect the face to the voice. He's heard her voice for eight or nine weeks or longer and when he goes onto the breast, he remembers that voice because he's heard it so often. And shortly therafter, he knows her face, he knows what she looks like by connecting the face, the voice and the smell. It's quite a remarkable thing, the rapid identification that he makes with the mother.

And in the first 45 minutes, the baby has a long, long period of the quiet alert state where he looks at the mother. He looks right at her. And this special state is the learning state. There's much to begin life looking at your mother. And so we think that the baby belongs with the father and the mother in the same bed as she delivered in at home or in a bed where the mother can be alone with her husband and take in the baby. This is especially good as a bonding time. The mother and father inspect the baby. And maybe they had wanted a boy and they imagined that he would have lots of hair and he would be smiling and they got a serious little girl with no hair at all. And they're taken by surprise. It takes a while for the baby to grow on them; maybe an hour or two, or maybe five, six days. Each parent is different. Some mothers say that they're bonded immediately. We think this is true for a certain kind of bonding, but after they've nursed for several days, they become intensely bonded to the baby. At this time they would not allow anybody they didn't know to touch their baby. And they would hurt anybody or kill anybody that would touch the baby. And that's a private feeling. And I say, that when they are not allowing anybody they don't know to touch their baby, that's the time that I think they're bonded.

Marshall Klaus, M.D. from *THE FIRST HOUR OF LIFE*

B

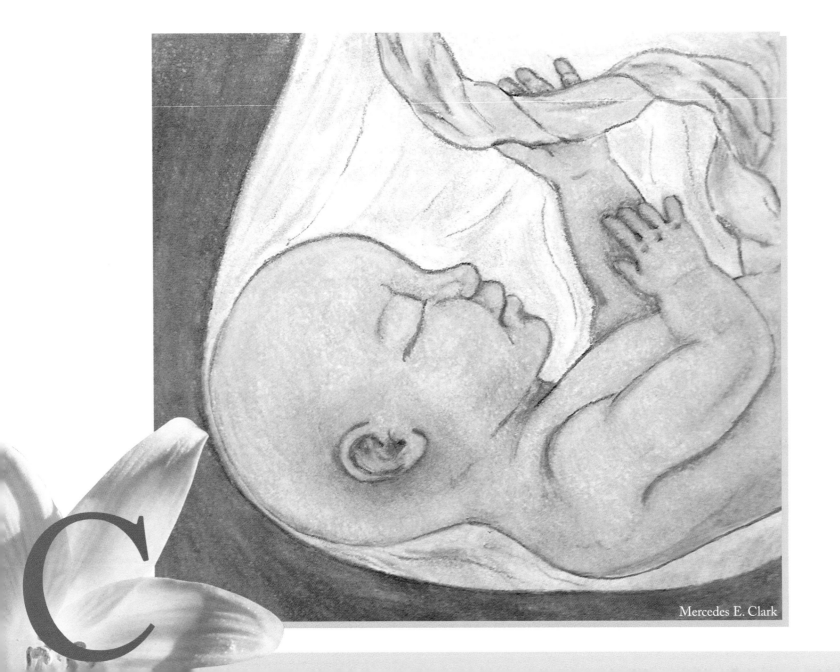

Mercedes E. Clark

Cord

My umbilical cord is the only thing I have touched besides myself these last months inside my womb-home. My cord and I drift together in this warm water. When I move, my cord follows me. When Mama laughs, my cord and I jiggle too. If I hold my cord with my hand, I can feel my own pulse! My cord is creamy white with blue vessels spiraling towards my placenta at the other end, ever so beautiful. Because of my cord, I am well nourished, and I am oxygen rich without breathing until...well, until I break through to the other side and drink exquisite air into my lungs! I cannot see or smell Mama yet, but we are connected by my cord, which spreads out like roots in the fertile soil of bearth.

- Deborah Allen, Midwife

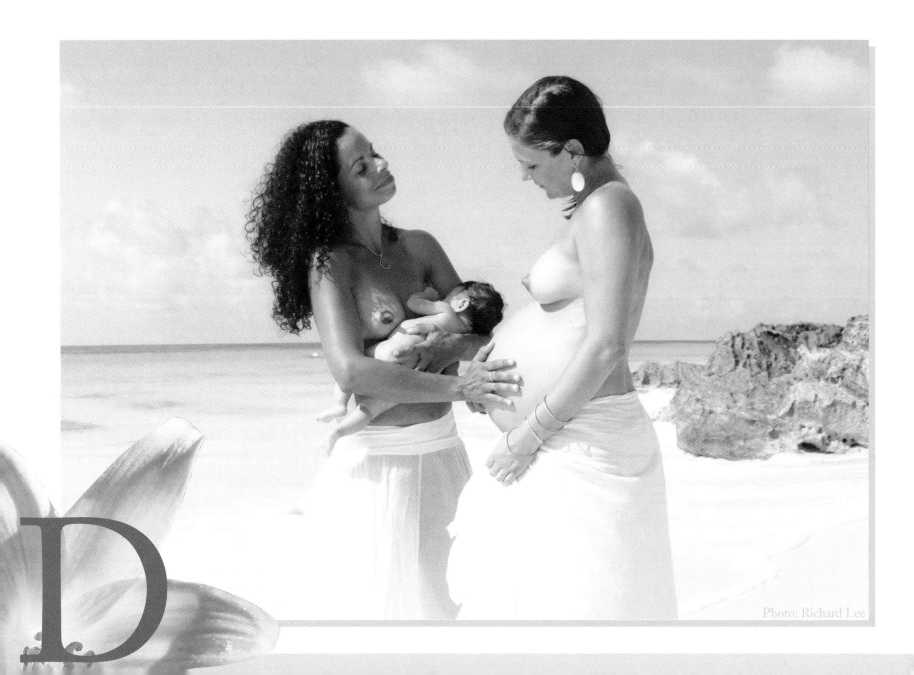

D

Deborah's Tenets

Deborah Allen and I once spent a long afternoon discussing just what we should put on our list of suggested supplies to give expectant moms. At the end of the day it read:

Home Birth Supplies
All you really need is love and a piece of cloth

A few items were suggested but there is no need to complicate birth with a lot of unnecessary "things" or interventions. The truth is, the more simple and fear free, the better. The optimum is for everyone to feel touched by the divine.

Deborah offers these Tenets for Birth to keep what is important at the forefront:
1. Birth is to be respected as a woman's private sexual and spiritual experience.
2. The birthing woman is steward of the birth of her child.
3. Life's design cannot be improved upon. Therefore birth, intelligently and exquisitly designed, is natural for mother and baby and cannot be improved upon.
4. Only those invited by the birthing woman shall attend the birth.
5. Only those actions requested by the birthing woman shall be done for her.
6. The mother and baby need each other before, during and after the birth and shall remain together. Their relationship is to be protected and cherished for it is our model of love.
7. We bring safety into the birth environment through our awareness of the presence of love, infinite and supreme.

D

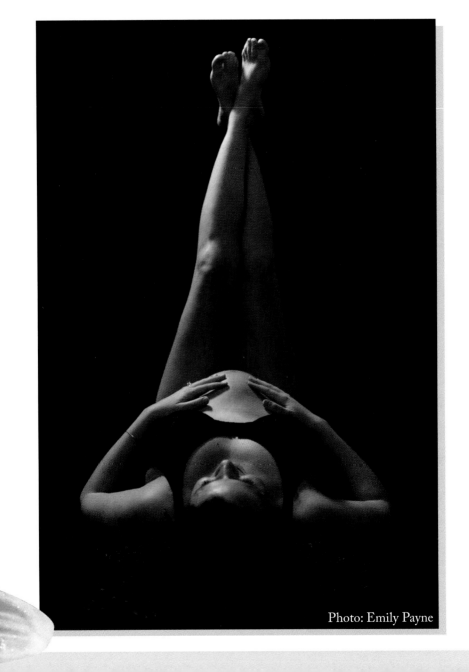

Photo: Emily Payne

Expecting

Body wiggles, eye contact and sometimes lots of sound are the newborn's way of communicating what is expected.

And before birth? The baby is already enjoying exquisite and complete womb service. What more might he expect?

Ina May Gaskin tells the story of a pregnant woman who was told that her babe in utero was deformed. Although the mother decided to keep her child, she was sad and depressed throughout the pregnancy. When the baby arrived, however, no abnormalities were found. The tests were mistaken. What a joy. But instead of the baby looking out in wonder at his new world, he arrived looking profoundly sad.

We know that a pregnant mother and her baby is a dyad. They are at one physically. But it may be that they are emotionally at one also. If that is the case, let mothers and babies hear only good stories and expect only the best. Because the very best Mother Nature has to offer… is on its way.

E

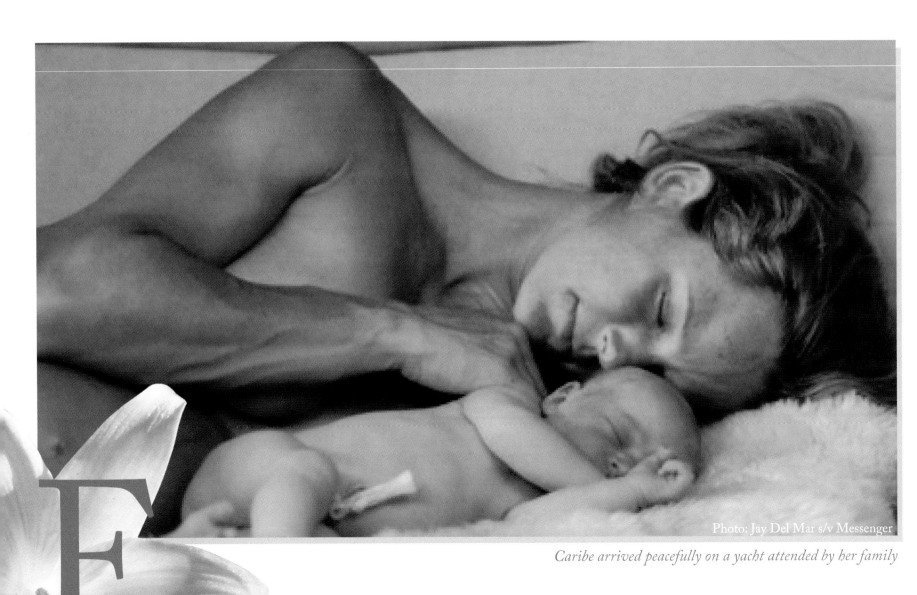

Photo: Jay Del Mar s/v Messenger

Caribe arrived peacefully on a yacht attended by her family

"The first great commandment is, don't let them scare you."
- *Elmer Davis*

The ability to enjoy birth, even experience its freedom and bliss, is tied to the ability to remove fear. Love, of course, is the strongest ally in removing fear. So to prepare women for childbirth, I would encourage mothers to go deeper into their spiritual practice, challenge their fears and increase their faith.

When I was nine months pregnant with our third child, I couldn't sleep at night. Finally, a friend said, "Sleeplessness is usually caused by fear." I didn't think I was afraid of anything but at his suggestion I sat down and examined my thoughts. It took about two hours before I discovered a latent fear of death.

This fear went back to my first visit with the midwife when she found a tumor. It was probably due to birth hormones, she said. "It'll go away when the baby arrives." What a shock. But then the midwife was so nonchalant and I was so busy with two little boys, I just forgot about it.

Subconsciously, however, the suggestion played out dramatically as danger and death. No wonder I couldn't sleep. When the fear was exposed, however, I could remove it with prayer, affirmation, and reason. I remember laughing at the suggestion of death in the face of this brilliant new life. With the fear gone, I slept like a baby and a few days later our little girl arrived.

F

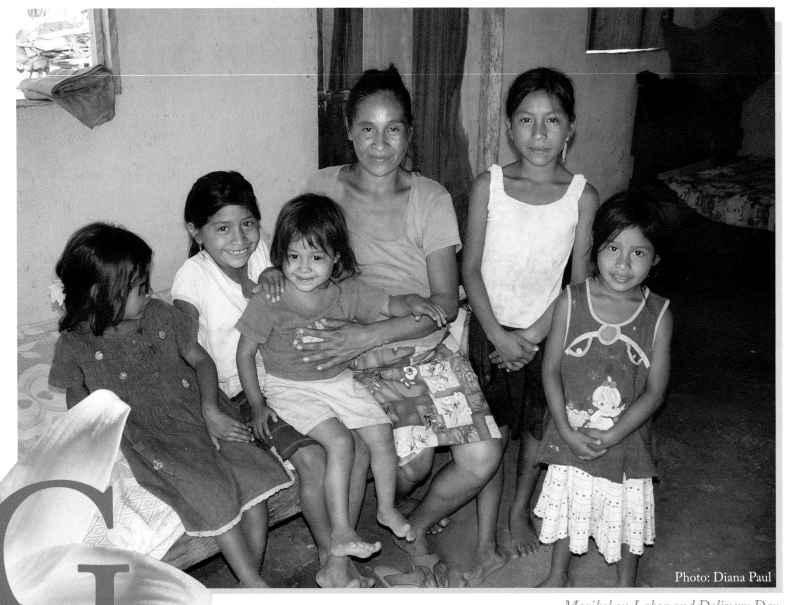

G

Maribel on Labor and Delivery Day

Grace

Mingo, Maribel and their children live without electricity or running water in a one-room house with a hard dirt floor. When they learned about the enormous number of women giving birth by cesarean section, they eagerly demonstrated their way. Maribel dropped to her knees and Mingo squatted in front of her. She pressed her forehead into his chest and he wrapped his arms around her waist. "See, like this," he said convincingly.

Mingo was proud to say that he caught three of his children before the midwife arrived. And Maribel was glad to have the birth of their ninth child filmed to show women that they needn't be afraid. Grace is uncomplicated. Both birth and grace proceed from the divine and profoundly affect the heart.

G

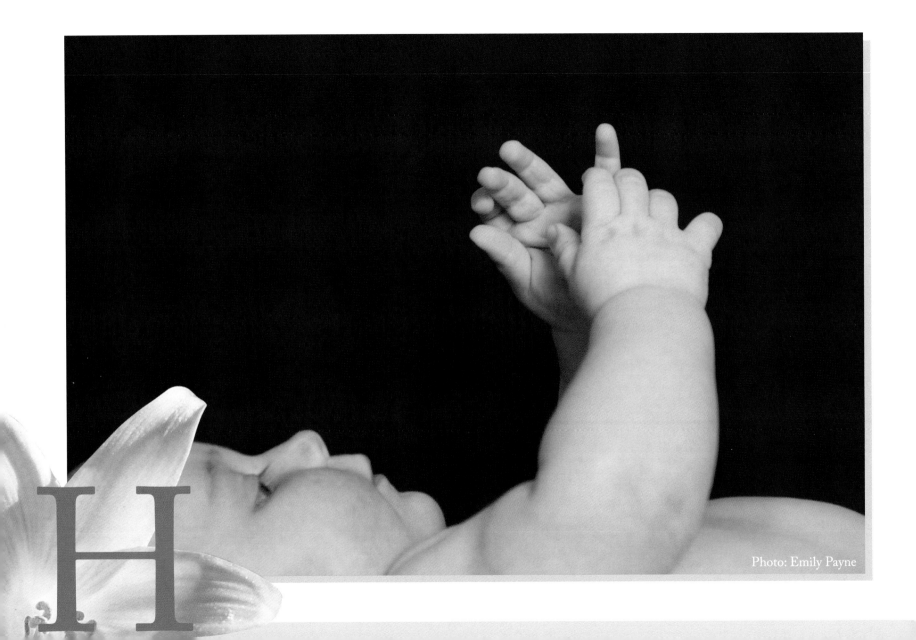

H.

HEAVEN. Now there's a thought.

Nothing has ever been able, ultimately, to convince me we live anywhere else.
And the heaven, more a verb than a noun, more a condition than a place,
Is all about leading with the heart in whatever broken or ragged state it's in,
Stumbling forward in faith until, from time to time, we miraculously
Find our way.

Our way to forgiveness, our way to letting go, our way to
understanding, compassion and peace.

It is laughter, I think that bubbles up at last and says, "I lo, I think we are there." And that "there"
is always here.

– Alice Walker

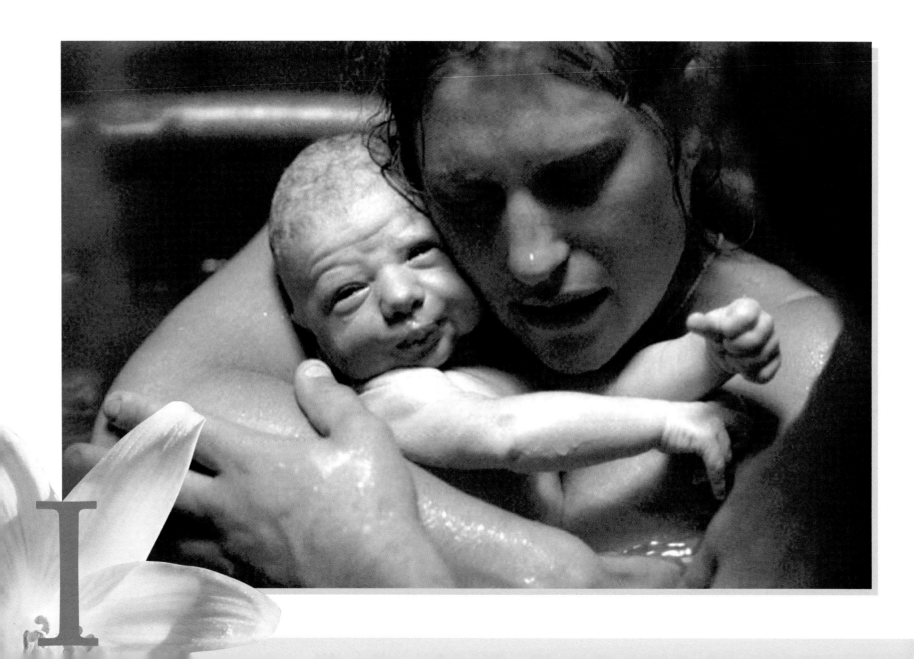

I

Instinct

After attending over a thousand births each, three homebirth midwives from three different continents said they had come to believe that birth, largely treated as a physical event, is really 80 - 90% psychological or spiritual.

I like to think that every laboring woman is given a sacred "how to" birth script. It is her script alone. She reads it by instinct. This leads her to that wild mix of surrender and power followed by the sudden, surprising and blissful moment of holding her own baby.

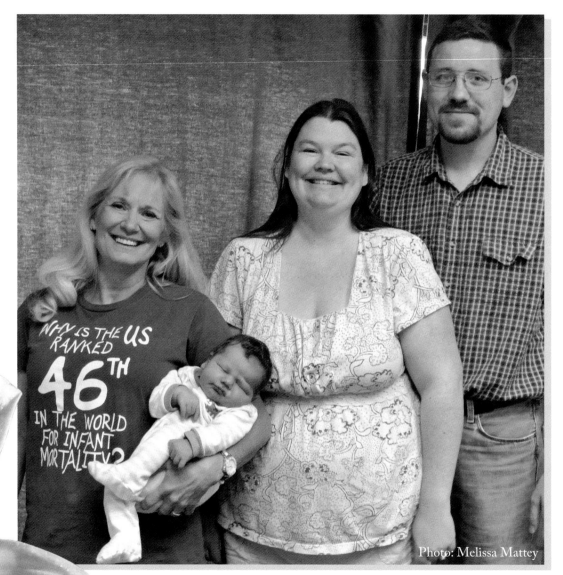

J

Homebirth Midwife Susan Gill holding baby Jack who weighed 12lbs 6oz. at birth. Marisa and Scott are smiling because Jack's older brother was smaller and arrived by caesarean section in the hospital ~ The obstetricians thought there was no other way

Photo: Melissa Mattey

"There's this factor called data. You can be the most prestigious scientist with a hypothesis but if the data conflicts with it, then you have to humbly accept that you're wrong. Another thing science has is this standard that you always have to compare with. It isn't just a matter of opinion."
- *Dr. Laurance Doyle, Astrophysicist*

"I am a medical doctor and a trained neonatalogist which means a pediatrician who specializes in the care of newborn babies. And I am also a reproductive scientist which means that after all of my training as a physician, I went back to the university to learn how to become a scientist. And that's important because what many people do not understand is, doctors are not scientists. And in fact, one of the biggest problems we have today in the care of women during pregnancy and birth is that there is a huge gap between what the doctors in the hospitals are doing and what we know scientifically to be the most important and best thing to do."
"Having a highly trained obstetrical surgeon attend a normal birth is analogous to having a pediatric surgeon babysit a healthy 2-year-old."
- *Dr. Marsden Wagner*

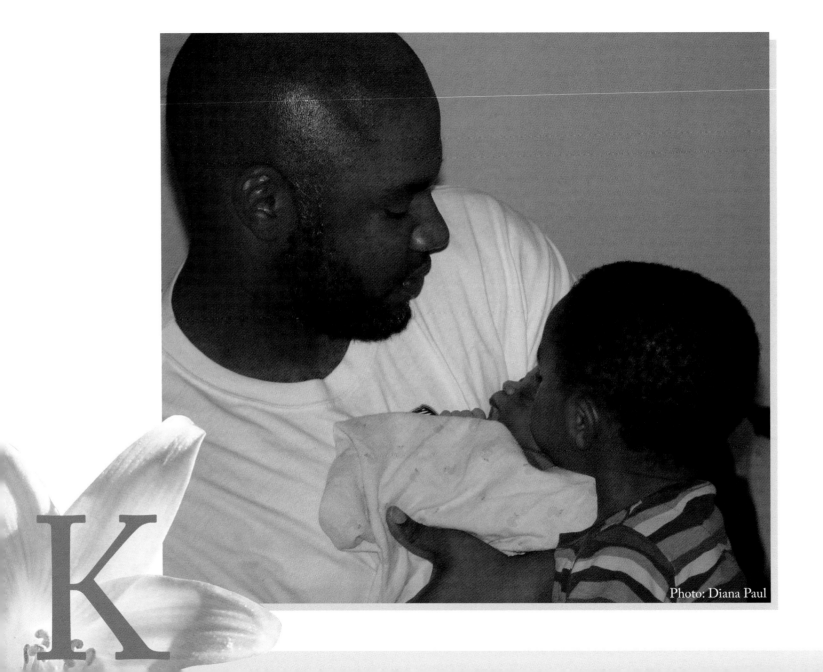

Photo: Diana Paul

K

Kindness

"They'll know how to birth. Give 'em love and kind words. That beats it all."
- *Margaret Charles Smith, Midwife*

"In former times, the emotional health of the pregnant woman was the job of all in her community, because it was understood a mother's attitude contributes greatly to her baby's health. It was traditional in other societies to protect a pregnant woman from hearing bad news. Also, it was said you should never argue with a pregnant woman. But if you ever do, give her the last word! In the old days in Japan, women practiced Taikyo, or "womb training," a form of prenatal attention to the mother's mental and spiritual health. In my practice as a midwife, I plead with my clients to stand guard at the doorway of their thinking, to dwell only on those thoughts that are encouraging and peaceful, to end conversations with people who are afraid of birth."
- *Deborah Allen, Midwife*

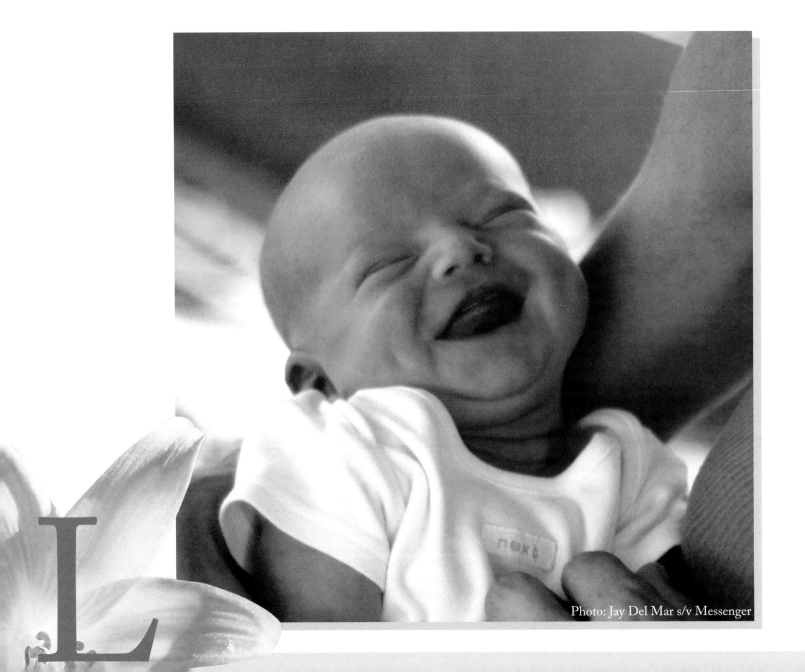

Photo: Jay Del Mar s/v Messenger

L

LAUGH *your baby out!*

Babies love laughter. It creates oxytocin, the 'happy hormone,' which, among other lovely uses, stimulates labor. Making the belly laugh, the mouth smile, the soul happy, is wonderful - especially when you're pregnant. Ina May Gaskin tells midwives, "If your lady is having a long labor, try asking her to smile. If the difficulty persists, ask her to smile broader. It is impossible to have a tight sphincter and smile at the same time."

The evening before our second child was born, I happened to watch a Flip Wilson rerun on Comedy Central. I could see and feel the baby moving all around as I shook with laughter.

Later that night, 2:30am to be exact, I got up and took a shower. I washed my hair, scrubbed the bathroom tile and wondered if what I was feeling might be false labor. At 3:15am I went back to bed but was immediately propelled out again by a powerful contraction. It was our baby arriving ahead of schedule to see what all the laughter was about. Thanks to Flip Wilson, my body must have been flooded with oxytocin, so I was only aware of being in labor for 7 ½ minutes. Thirty years later, this baby does a great Flip Wilson imitation.

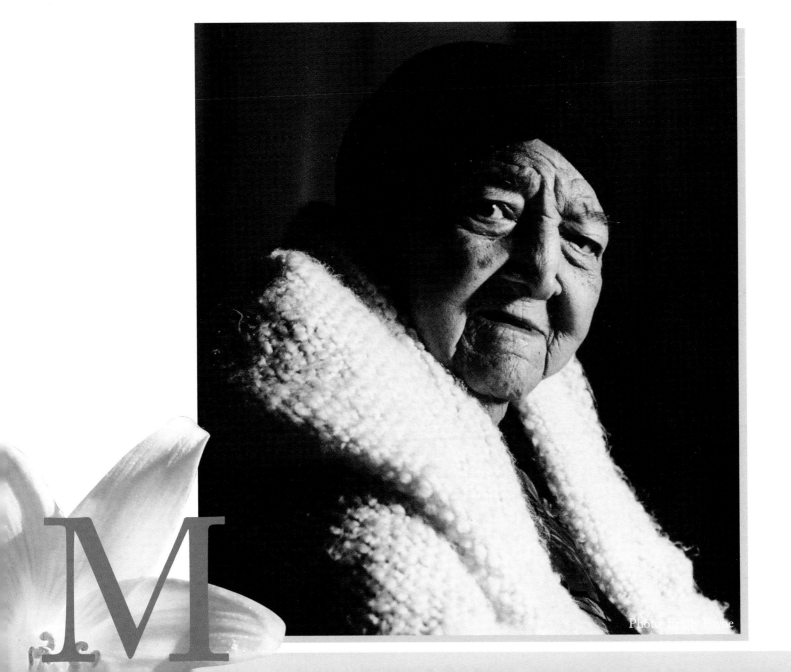

Photo: Emily Payne

M

Miss Margaret

The Granny System was a legal, necessary and proud part of the South before, during and after segregation. Thousands of licensed and experienced Granny Midwives attended hundreds of thousands of births. In 1976, however, Alabama outlawed the Granny System and families lost a legitimate and cost effective choice for birth.

One story Margarent Charles Smith tells from her legendary career as an Alabama Granny Midwife demonstrates the obstacles she had to overcome and the passion with which she served her community. Miss Margaret tried to take a laboring woman with eclampsia to the local hospital but the all-white facility refused to take the woman in. "She might die!" Miss Margaret pleaded. The doctor replied, "That's not my problem," and sent them away.

Although the woman was unconscious, her labor continued and the baby was born in the taxi. The driver took the three of them to Miss Margaret's house where she cared for the mother until she was able to care for her baby. In over 3,500 home births, Miss Margaret never lost a mother.

M

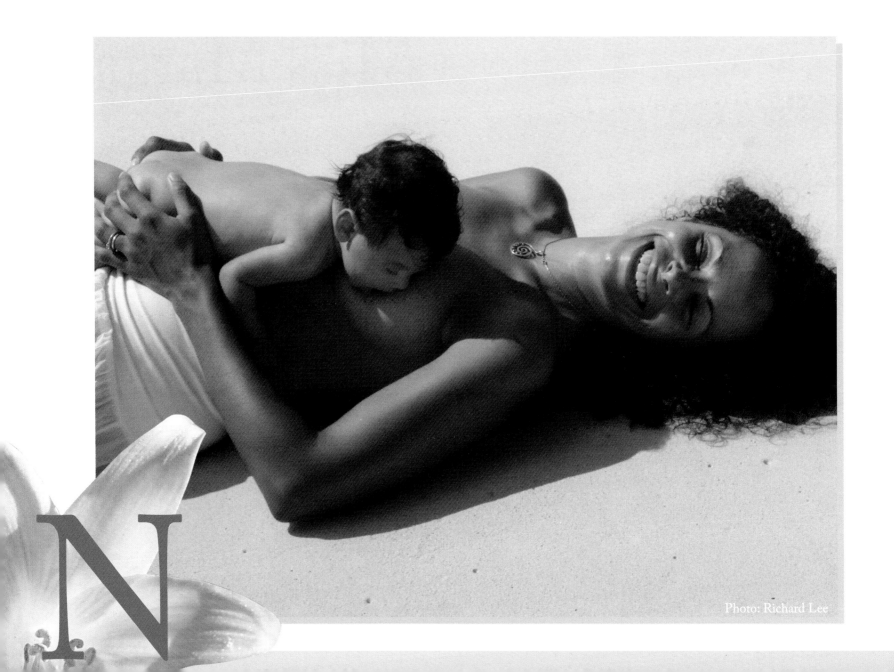

N

Nursing

The baby's first meal comes as warm, golden droplets of colostrom. Intense joy, cuddling, suckling, the sound of her baby's cry are all emotional states which call down this sweet nectar. For the first few days, colostrom nourishes and establishes the baby's immune system. Then the breasts fill with milk and a long period of luxurious nursing follows.

Operating on the highest principle of supply and demand, produced by the stimulus of love, it is a mistake to think that colostrum or breast milk can in any way be imitated or manufactured.

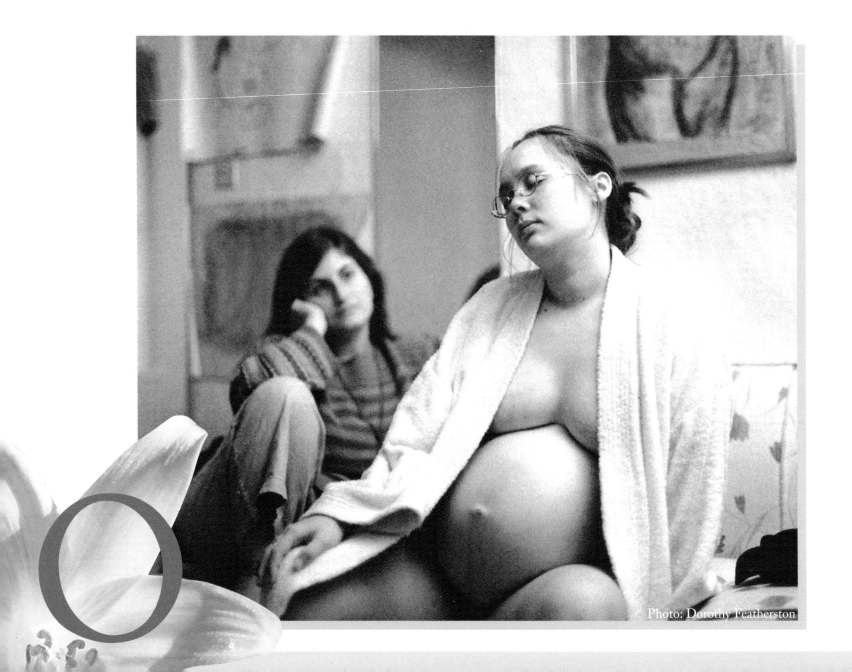

A laboring woman's first need is to feel secure and to have privacy, not to feel observed. In fact, laboring women need to be protected against any sort of useless stimulation. They need to feel free, spontaneous, not to have read too many books. When they just do what they feel during labor, they find a posture which helps them to isolate themselves. For example, you find women on hands and knees as if praying. To pray is to reduce the activity of the intellect so you can reach another reality of space and time. It is exactly what laboring women need to cut themselves off from the world, to go to another planet. When women are giving birth by themselves without any medication, there is a time when they are as if on another planet. That means that they are reducing the activity of the intellect. So women, when they are not guided, when they don't feel observed, when there are not people around watching them…spontaneously find postures which make sense, which help them to release the necessary hormones.

- *Dr. Michel Odent*

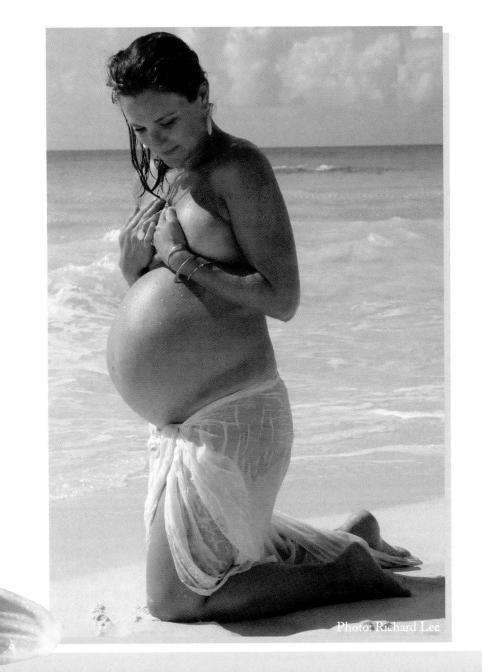

Photo: Richard Lee

P

Birth itself is a prayer.   Self-surrender, gentleness, strength, trust and purity are its requirements. When we were interviewing midwives, the cameraman would ask, "What are the five things you would tell a pregnant woman to prepare her for birth?" A French Canadian midwife, Celine LeMay, replied, "I don't prepare people for birth. Why would you prepare for a baby? It's well done for a million years."

The cameraman persisted, "But what would you tell a woman…"

Celine: "I would say go into the forest and be one with nature, it will help you more than reading books or classes."

Cameraman again: "But what if…"

Celine again with a rich French accent: "Read poems, pray, sing, dance, feel and listen.   I'm not the expert! I'm just a tool. A woman needs to be connected with her own truth."

"Be still and know that I am God." ~ Psalms 46:1

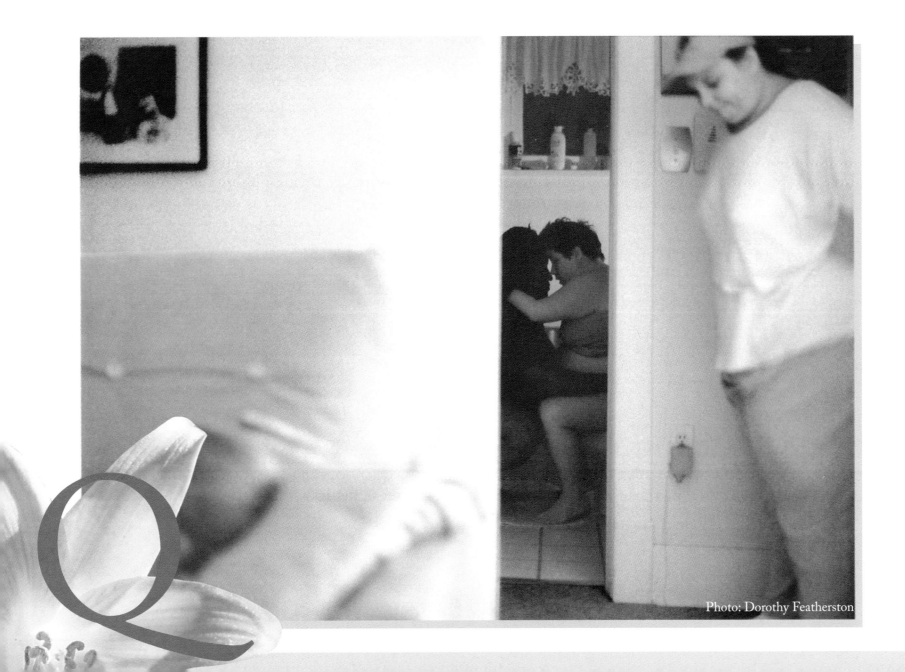

Photo: Dorothy Featherston

Just before she married, a friend confessed that she was afraid of birth. "Hmm," I said. "Why don't you watch Birth Day?" Eleven minutes later after watching this powerful video, Lizzy said, "I think I'm healed!"

Later when Lizzy was pregnant, she followed this advice: When you think you might be in labor...
1.   Go for a long walk. If you still think you are in labor...
2.   Go out to dinner and follow dinner with
3.   A late night movie.
This routine has the wonderful effect of quieting anxiety, distracting the mind and relaxing the body. Then the cervix can open.

Lizzy timed her contractions in the theater and finally whispered, "I think we should go home now." She called her midwife on the way and asked her to meet them at the house. But as soon as they got home and the door was closed, Lizzy felt the urge to push. Her husband knelt down next to her and caught their baby. The midwife arrived soon thereafter and helped settle everyone in. Lizzy went from fear to triumph and now loves to share how she was transformed by birth.

Shh, women need deep quiet so they can hear their own instincts.

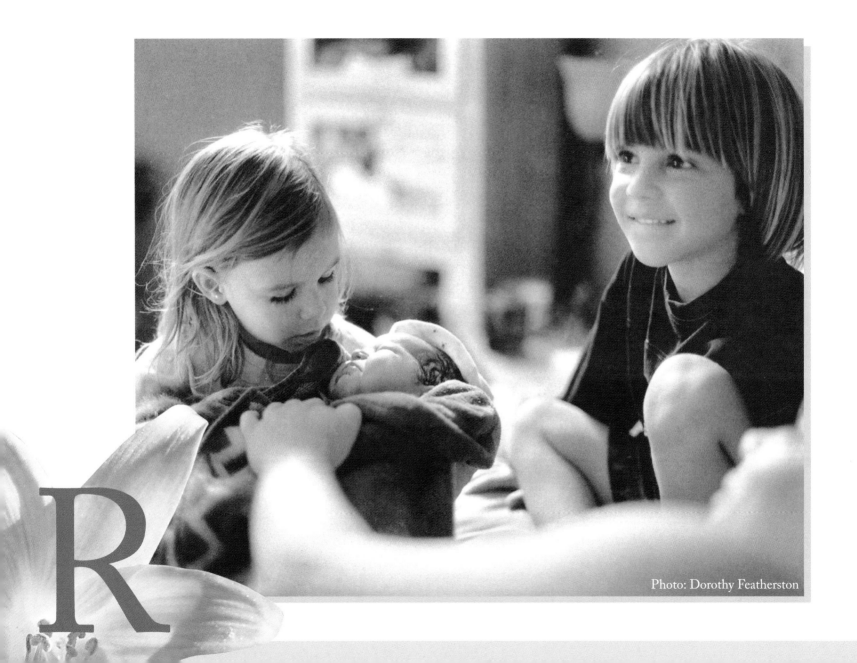

R

Photo: Dorothy Featherston

Receiving

"Every good gift and every perfect gift comes from above." ~ James 1:17

Deborah and I attended a homebirth where the mom and dad had thought of every last detail. Even the neighbors had assigned tasks: Measuring the temperature of the room and the birthing tub, taking care of the baby's sister, making casseroles, etc. Yet when the baby arrived in this perfectly loving and thoughtful atmosphere, he cried and cried and cried. Instinctively, we all started singing a song his sister had been singing and dancing to during the pregnancy. The baby stopped crying immediately and looked around the room with wide open eyes. Through music his surroundings became familiar and he was able to receive the warmth and love his parents were waiting to give.

After the unspeakably beautiful birth of our first child, I knew I could be even more fearless and therefore more helpful to the baby the next time I gave birth. Confidently following my instincts even more closely, I was led to give birth on my knees ~ literally. The next two babies loved this relaxed and prayerful position that allowed them to slip out in minutes, not hours.

R

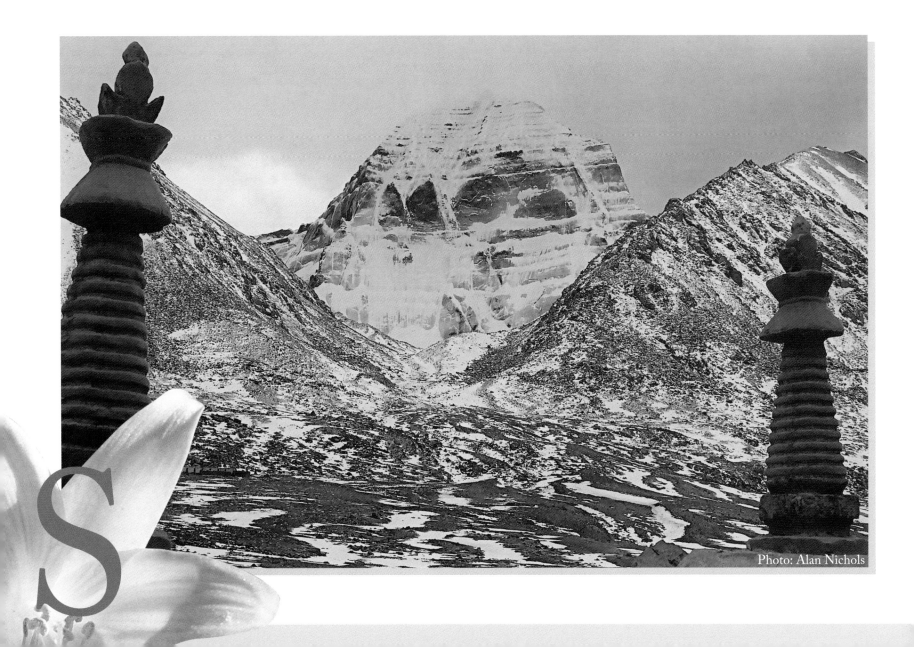

S

Photo: Alan Nichols

Sacred

Why is Mount Kailash recognized as the most sacred mountain in the world and what does that have to do with birth?

Thousands of Buddhist, Hindu, Jain and Bonpo pilgrims walk around its base each year. They say no one has ever set foot on the mountain itself because that would be sacrilegious. Here she looks like a baby emerging from her mother's womb.

Could this similarity be what makes her so sacred? Are not those who attend birth like pilgrims journeying to a sacred place?

S

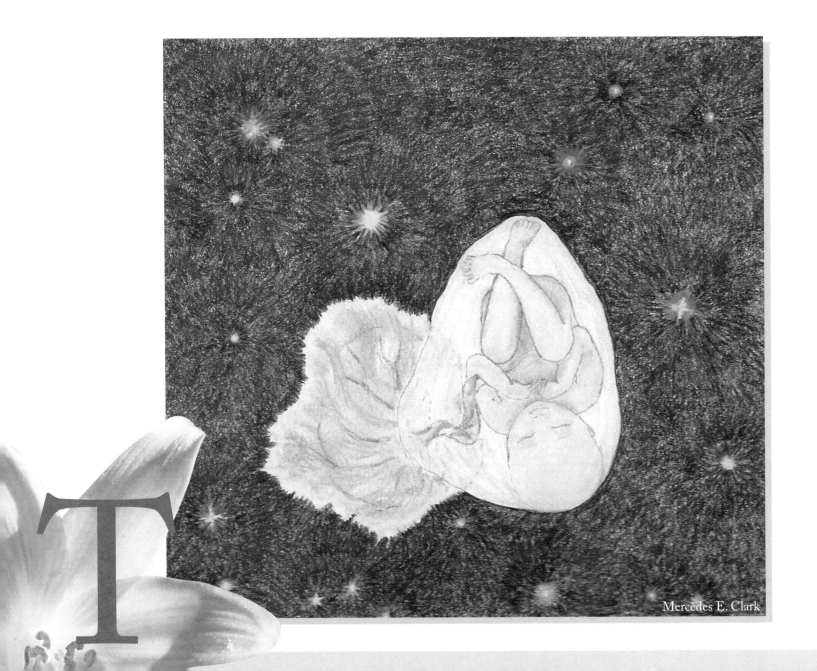

Mercedes E. Clark

T

Sputnik was the word on everyone's lips in 1957. It was the first satellite to orbit the earth. In 1961, Yuri Gagarin, a Russian astronaut, became the first human being to orbit the earth. The Americans quickly followed with Alan Shepherd, John Glenn and others. These early travelers were launched into space and came home to a world crazy with excitement about their achievement.

What is it the astronauts did again?

1. They were carried by the Mothership to a place unknown.
2. They experienced, quiet, weightlessness and confinement.
3. When they arrived, they saw an entirely new world.

Just like Mother Nature's cosmic and inscrutable Transportation System for birth.

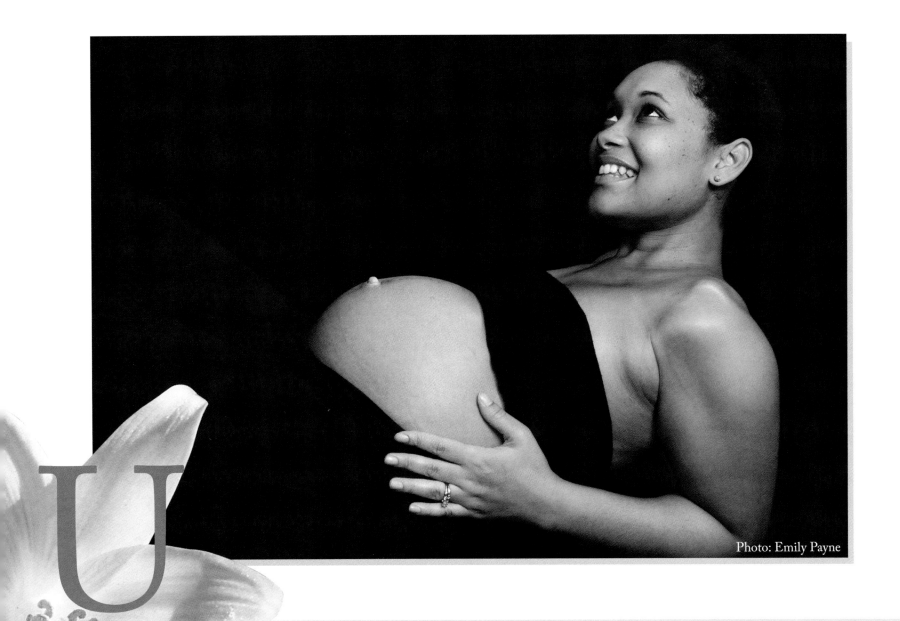

U

I asked astrophysicist, Dr. Laurance Doyle, "How unique are we in the universe?"

He replied, "By 'we' you mean our planet, species, individuals? In detail our planet is certainly unique on any scale we can practically consider. But generally, I think of life as a field expressing itself everywhere rather than a particle like a person, a fly or plant for example. And the processes that lead to a habitable planet can go on in billions of other places in our galaxy which is just one of trillions of galaxies. As a species, we seem to be the first on this planet to develop, for example, space travel – this is quite an original.

"Being a fraternal triplet myself, my folks emphasized individuality. So I see that as the first quality in every person as well. To me, the foundation of our value to each other – our first precious attribute – is our uniqueness in the universe."

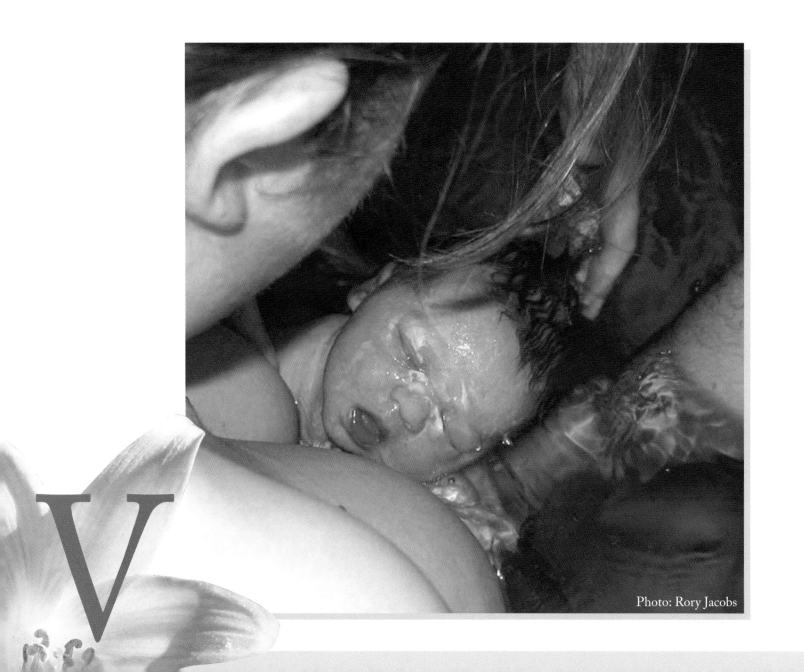

Photo: Rory Jacobs

VBAC

SEPARATED
(For Finnn, my first baby who was born via c-section)

When they said they had to take you then
The thought of holding you saw me through
Just a span of an hour and a blade separated us

Your first night I kept you in my arms
And every night ever after that
Just whispery fractions of cloth separated us

During baths the pair of us cuddle and splash
And remember back to still warmer times before us
Just rhythmic waters of the future separated us

The first signs of the softness of your touch amaze
Your curious and tender holds make me your captive
Just skin printed like mine and tiny toes separated us

Your brilliant babble explains the unexplainable
Constant and bleating and dearest in tone
Just mirrored sounds said softly separated us

As you near two, all proud rolls and hand stands
Thoughts of times without you get fuzzier but one
Just the knowing that nothing really separated us

JOINED
(For little lady Beatrix, my second baby and first girl born
VBAC at home in water)

Take two was going to be different
Water and warmth and no hospitals at all
We were joined from the start, and going to stay that way

We went against the odds and the expected
Doctors disowned and tried to scare us silly
But on we went naturally, joined in our own time

There were no ruptures or worries or deadlines
Just endless walks up familiar stairs 36 hours long
Blizzarded in we joined the quiet of a waiting world

Midwife and husband and child then baby came
And the promise I would know you well enough
To lift you from the water myself, joined us

Caroline Schaefer-Hills

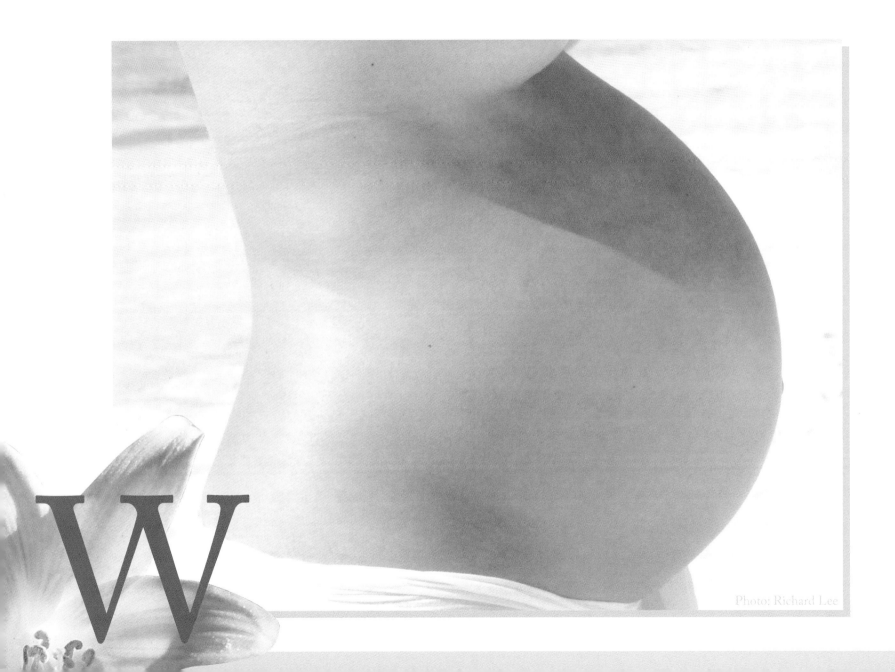

W

Liquid oceans throw sparkling diamonds to the sun and moonbeams to the stars. They entertain giant vessels, sea creatures and surfers alike. An ocean is a magnificent playground, an uncompromising power.
It is feminine – a pregnant womb rocking its secret treasure.

ROCKING

The sea rocks her thousands of waves.
The sea is divine.
Hearing the loving sea
I rock my son.

The wind wandering by night
Rocks the wheat.
Hearing the loving wind
I rock my son.

God, the Father, soundlessly rocks
His thousands of worlds.
Feeling His Hand in the shadow
I rock my son.

- Gabriela Mistral

My 85 year old neighbor went down to the harbor every day. He took a nap on his little boat – the "Salty Dog."
When he returned, he always looked younger, happier. It was his womb experience he said.

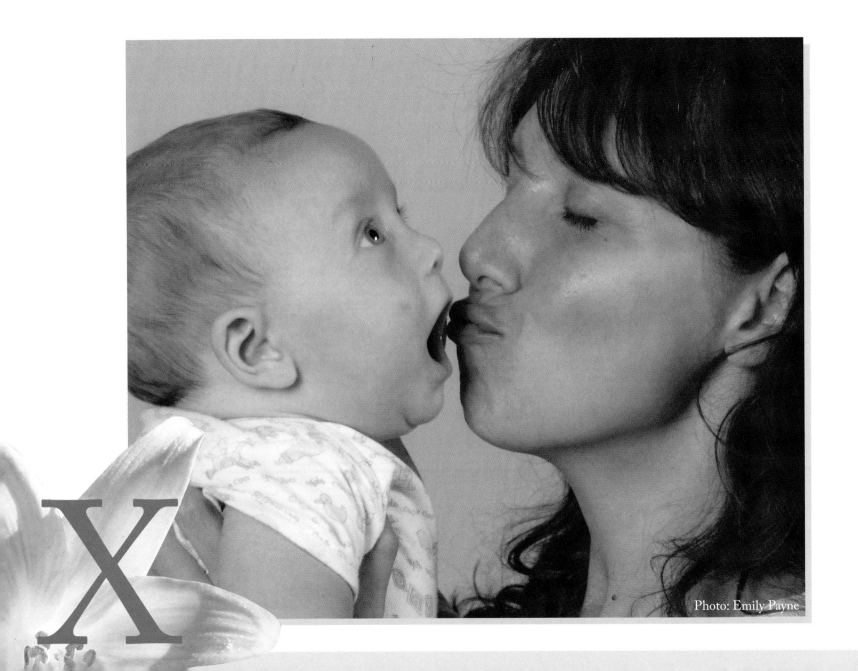

X

And the meaning is?

○ Abbreviation for Executive Officer

○ Abbreviation for Kiss and Hug

○ The first move in making a baby

○ What the world needs now

○ All of the above

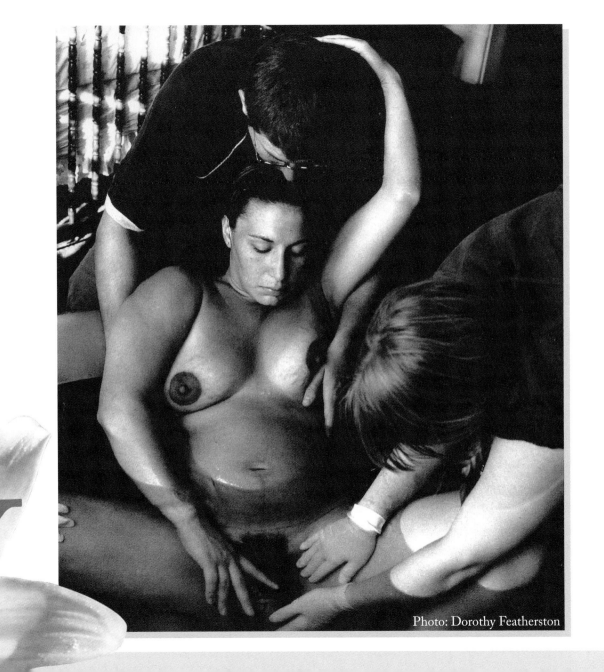

Y

Photo: Dorothy Featherston

Yin Yang

This beautiful picture evokes the essence of yin yang as the woman's arms curl up and down in the shape of the ancient Chinese symbol. One hand reaches for her husband, and the other for her baby.

Yin, when combined with Yang, gives birth to all that comes to be. One aspect of yin yang is that of man and woman coming together in balance. Here it culminates in deep concentration and opening in the woman as she gives birth.

- Serena Eastman

Y

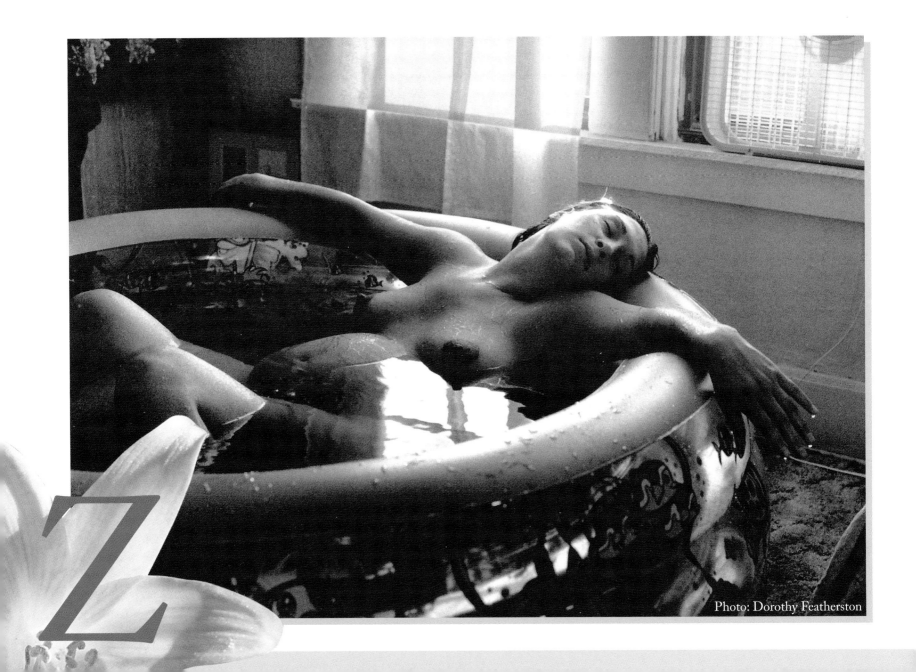

Z

Zone

Being in the 'zone' refers to experiencing peak performance. The body, nimble and obedient, plays second fiddle to the mind.

A woman in the birth zone has completely surrendered to the process. She is in babyland as some midwives describe it.

If you are fortunate enough to see her there, don't ask anything of her. Just quietly admire her and breathe. Don't be afraid if she cries out, trust that her soul is guiding. Don't distract her. Rather, show her your love with an absolute confidence in her ability to give birth. She can do it. She is giving birth to her baby.

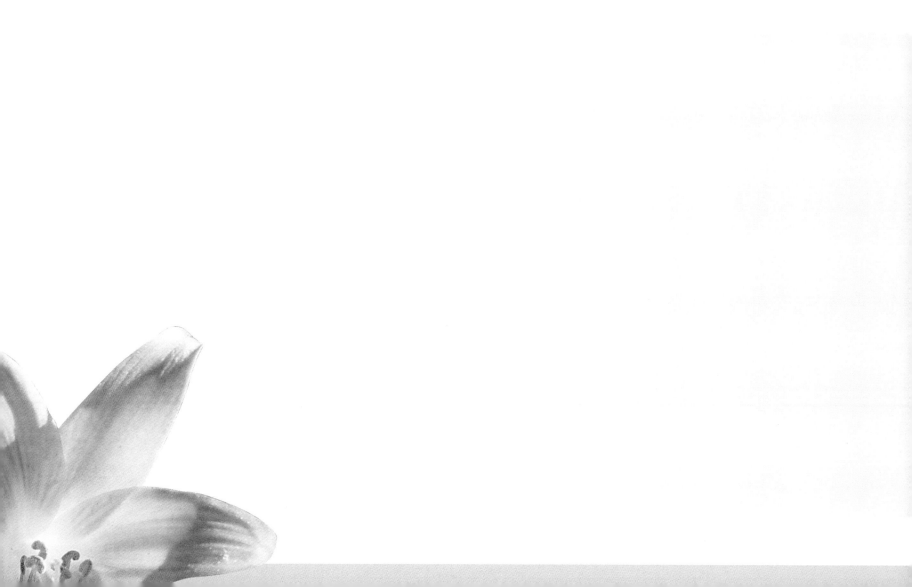

About the Author

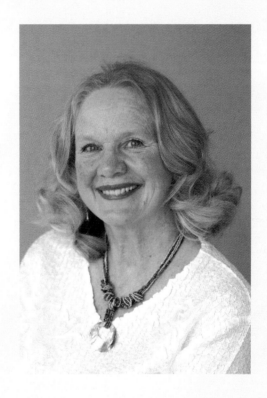

Diana Paul graduated from Sonoma State University during the Vietnam War. It was a time of campus disruption, confusion and convocations. It was also a time of independent investigation and experimentation. And so it was, in a spacious campus hallway at Sonoma State that she first saw a movie depicting natural birth. The couple screening the film had just given birth and delighted in sharing their new baby and every possible detail of their birth experience.

Years later, Diana learned that her husband had been born at home with an immigrant doctor attending. And her husband's father was born on Catalina Island with only his parents attending. The doctor missed the boat and the birth. Before that, everyone in his family was born at home with or without a midwife or doctor attending.

Knowledge of this history gave Diana inspiration to choose the same simple way for the births of her three children. The first two arrived at home in Mill Valley and the last at her in-law's home in Oakland, California. The births were exhilarating, transforming and very different from one another. She wanted to share her experience but it was not the right time. Homebirth was considered unorthodox and downright scary.

After taking some nursing classes in San Francisco and a midwifery course in El Paso, her family moved to Massachusetts and she began attending homebirths with Deborah Allen. This was an eyeopening experience and so began her journey into midwifery and filming natural birth. Her first film, Birth Day, was installed in the Museum of Science in Boston.

In 1999, Diana founded Sage Femme Inc., a non-profit organization which later became Love Delivers. She has been the Executive Director since inception ~ producing films, creating festivals and overseeing events which highlight the benefits of natural, drug-free birth.

Glossary of Terms

Wild: Untamed, natural, free. A wilderness, a universe, a baby arriving on planet earth, a woman in labor: These are wild natural states with their own order, time and place. At birth, it takes mindfulness to let wild things be.

Naked: Unadulterated, pure, true. We want the Naked Truth. Who says that women are broken and their bodies can't give birth? The naked truth is women are made for this. Love, not fear, maintains and delivers both mother and baby. Believe the Naked Truth.

Ladies: *Consider the lilies of the field, how they grow: They labour not, neither do they spin…Matt 6:28.* Lilies and ladies come with everything necessary for splendid reproduction. Slipping into the wild, surrendering the outer garments of preconception, opinion and protocol, is what ladies giving birth do naturally.

46: Forty-six was the US ranking for infant mortality in 2011. By 2013, the US was ranked 50th among nations according to the CIA World Factbook. Why does the US have such poor outcomes for birth when it outspends every other country in the world on healthcare?

WHO: World Health Organization. WHO is an agency of the United Nations concerned with international public health including sexual and reproductive health. Studies and research by WHO have consistently shown that the best outcomes for women and babies occur when a country's cesarean section rate is between 5% and 10%. Rates above 15% appear more harmful than beneficial.

Caesarean Section: A caesarean section is major abdominal surgery to remove babies from the womb. It is the most common operation in the world and the most costly way to give birth. C-section rates vary from doctor to doctor, hospital to hospital and country to country. Typical, uncomplicated surgical births range in cost from $14,000 to $25,000 or more. Usually, the baby receives a separate bill. The baby's bill may be as low as $1,500 or as high as tens of thousands of dollars if she/he needs to go to the neonatal intensive care unit. These costs do not in any way reflect the emotional, spiritual and physical costs the mother and baby pay when they are separated at a surgical birth. By contrast, a typical midwife attended home or birth center delivery averages $2,000-$7,000 which often includes prenatal visits as well.

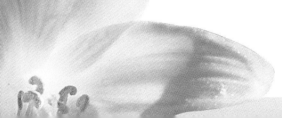

Amniotic Fluid: Inside the womb, a double membrane ~ "bag of waters" ~ surrounds the amniotic fluid in which the baby develops. Warm and spa-like, this nutrient rich amniotic fluid allows the baby to move safely and easily inside the sac. About a third of this sterile fluid is absorbed and replaced every hour. When the baby is born, the mother's nipples emit a powerful scent not unlike amniotic fluid. Instinctively sucking and smelling the fluid on his little hands, the baby is drawn by a similar smell from his mother's breasts. He then inches his way up from his mother's abdomen for his first meal out. This is called the breast crawl. Every healthy newborn can do this.

Colostrum: This is the baby's first meal. It is a yellowish liquid produced by the mother's breasts. Colostrum precedes breast milk for several days after birth. It flows on demand like breast milk. Colostrum is highly nutritive, notably in protein and calories. It is a key ingredient in establishing the baby's immune system as it contains antibodies and lymphocyte. Colostrum also acts as a laxative to clear the baby's bowel of meconium. Never underestimate the immense power and good that this nearly invisible nectar can achieve.

Uterine Contractions: This is the physical signal, like a whisper at first and then a shout, that the baby is coming.

Oxytocin ~ the 'love hormone': is released by the mother's body, contractions begin and eventually the baby arrives. The process can take from a few minutes to several days. To shorten the time or stress of labor, contractions should either be completely welcomed or completely ignored. Birth may be an involuntary act but contractions are related to the mother's ability to handle fear and manage suggestions of pain.

Eclampsia: Eclampsia is rarely seen where there is proper prenatal care and nutrition. It is an extreme metabolic imbalance in pregnancy.

Placenta: This word comes from the Latin word for cake. It is also called afterbirth. The placenta develops alongside the baby to provide constant nourishment. It is attached to the wall of the womb and connected to the baby by the umbilical cord. The placenta provides the mother and baby with hormones to promote lactation, prevent preterm labor, resist disease, and recycle waste, blood and oxygen.

VBAC: Many women choose a Vaginal Birth After Caesarean.

Without Whose Help WNL (the book) Would Not Be

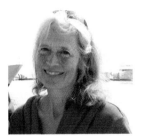

Deborah Allen, midwife
Cambridge, MA. USA

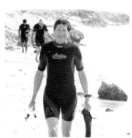

Daniel C. Bort, Esq.
San Francisco, CA

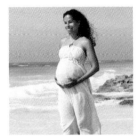

Sophia Cannonier-Watson,
Visionary Advisor, Bermuda

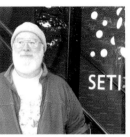

Dr. Laurance Doyle, SETI
Mountain View, CA

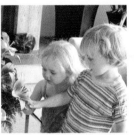

Beatrix & Finn Schaefer-Hills
Traverse City, MI

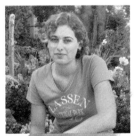

Mercedes E. Clark, Artist
Santa Rosa, CA

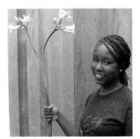

Brenda Vaxter,
Editor

Wendell Davis, Filmmaker
Frank Ferrel, Filmmaker
Dr. Michel Odent

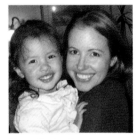

Erin Sutherland,
Graphic Designer

Ina May Gaskin, Midwife
Phyllis and Marshall Klaus
Celine LeMay, Midwife

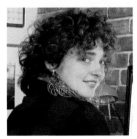

Serena Eastman,
Editor

Susan Scott Gill, Midwife
Danielle Centeno, Doula
Margaret Charles Smith, Midwife

Dr. Marsden Wagner

Alice Walker, Author

Jacquelyn Hadley, Editor

Christine DeCosta

Caroline Schaefer-Hills, Professor
Northwestern Michigan College
Creative Design Team:
  Emily Kane
  Jaymie Hatt
  Ashley Dansby

Acknowledgements

Photography Credits

Alan Nichols
Belvedere, USA

"The Sacred Mountain is the symbol of creation, of nations, of peoples, of religions and of the human spirit. The mountain joins heaven and earth to create Spirit as man joins woman to create 'persona spiritus.'"

Sacred Mountains have been Alan Nichol's world for 35 years.

Jay Del Mar s/v Messenger
Natasha Gonzalez Reece
Rory Jacobs
Melissa Mattey

Dorothy Featherston
Valdosta, GA. USA

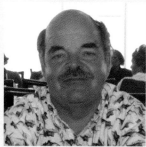

Richard Lee

Richard James Lee
Devonshire, Bermuda

The most beautiful gift God has blessed us with is making a human life, and there is nothing I enjoy more than taking photographs of a woman during her pregnancy, childbirth and nursing.

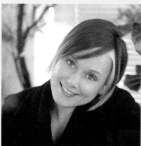

Emily Payne

Emily Payne
EP Images
San Francisco, CA
www.emilypayne.com

I am so proud and honored to be part of this project. Not having the experience of giving birth, I still value the love and care for a woman's body and baby during the intimate and gentle time of pregnancy.

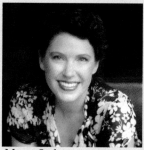

Megan Sachs

Megan Sachs Photography
www.megansachsphotography.com

Photographing pregnancy, birth and newborns is my passion. I cherish the opportunities I have to write life stories through my photographs. It brings me joy to capture the beauty of new life and document these fleeting moments for families to share with generations to come.

"What amazes me is that in a little more than a hundred years, the hospital birth, a process that sterilizes the experience and anesthetizes it's raw, primordial power, has become the norm and home birth the oddity in America. In fact, home birthing is illegal in some states and some insurance agencies will not cover it because a home birth is 'not a medical necessity'. When did hospitalization become a requirement for normal childbirth?" - Mike, my husband

These photos have come about as a result of the birth of our daughter, Hannah, and my need to heal some emotional wounds left by my hospital experience. Over the last four years it has become increasingly important to me to show that home birth is a safe and healthy alternative to the typical hospital experience of assembly line epidurals, scheduled C-sections, and other invasive procedures that strip the woman of her confidence as a mother. When a woman gives birth without interventions, she is empowered by her experience as the true depth of her physical and emotional reserves is revealed. At each birth my focus is on the mother and her support team because that is where the beauty and power manifest, and the miracle of childbirth begins. I've discovered that the range of women choosing home birth crosses all economic status and cultural boundaries. The one commonality is their desire for a more intimate and personal birthing experience.

Being Born Is Important
By Carl Sandburg

Being born is important
You who have stood at the bedposts
and seen a mother on her high harvest day,
the day of the most golden of harvest moons for her.

You who have seen the new wet child
dried behind the ears,
swaddled in soft fresh garments,
pursing its lips and sending a groping mouth
toward nipples where white milk is ready.

You who have seen this love's payday
of wild toiling and sweet agonizing.

You know being born is important.
You know that nothing else was ever so important to you.
You understand that the payday of love is so old,
So involved, so traced with circles of the moon,
So cunning with the secrets of the salts of the blood.
It must be older than the moon, older than salt.

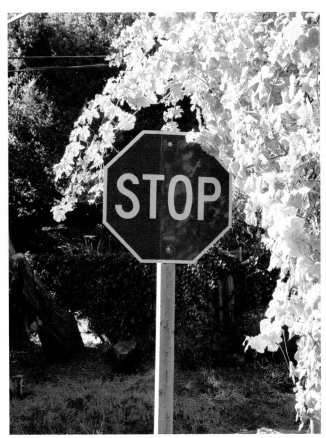

Stop sign at Las Lomas crowned with wild grape vine

It is my deepest desire that our species fall in love with Mother Nature again. Her design for birth is perfect. She does most of the work! There is very little that we women need to do beyond: Trust, follow our instincts, remove fear and exercise infinite patience. We give our babies the very best when we interfere the very least.

In peace and joy and power,

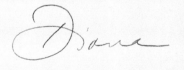

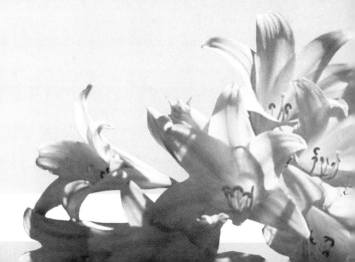